Gene Based Therapy for sicke cell(CASGEVY AND LYFGNIA)

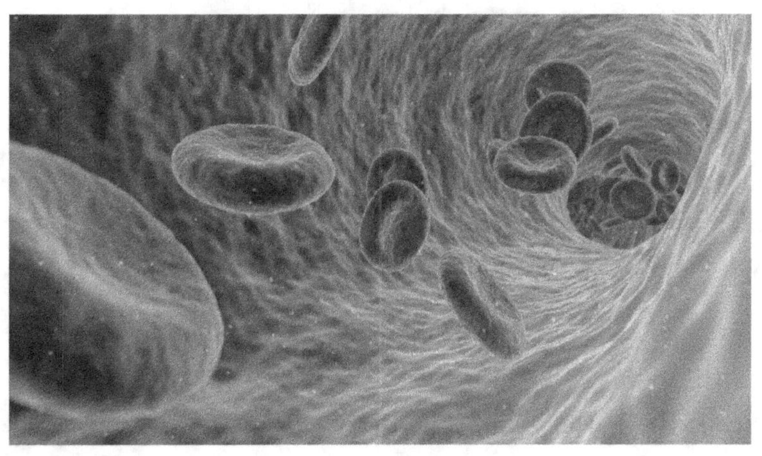

Transformative Gene-Based Therapies for Sickle Cell Disease

Richard William

Title: Gene-Based Therapy for Sickle Cell Disease

Subtitle: Unlocking the Potential: Transformative Gene-Based Therapies for Sickle Cell Disease
Author: Richard William

Publisher: Amazon

Cover Design: Richard William

Disclaimer: The information provided in this book is for educational and informational purposes only. It does not intend to replace professional medical advice or treatment. Readers are encouraged to consult with healthcare professionals for specific medical advice tailored to their individual conditions.

Table of Contents

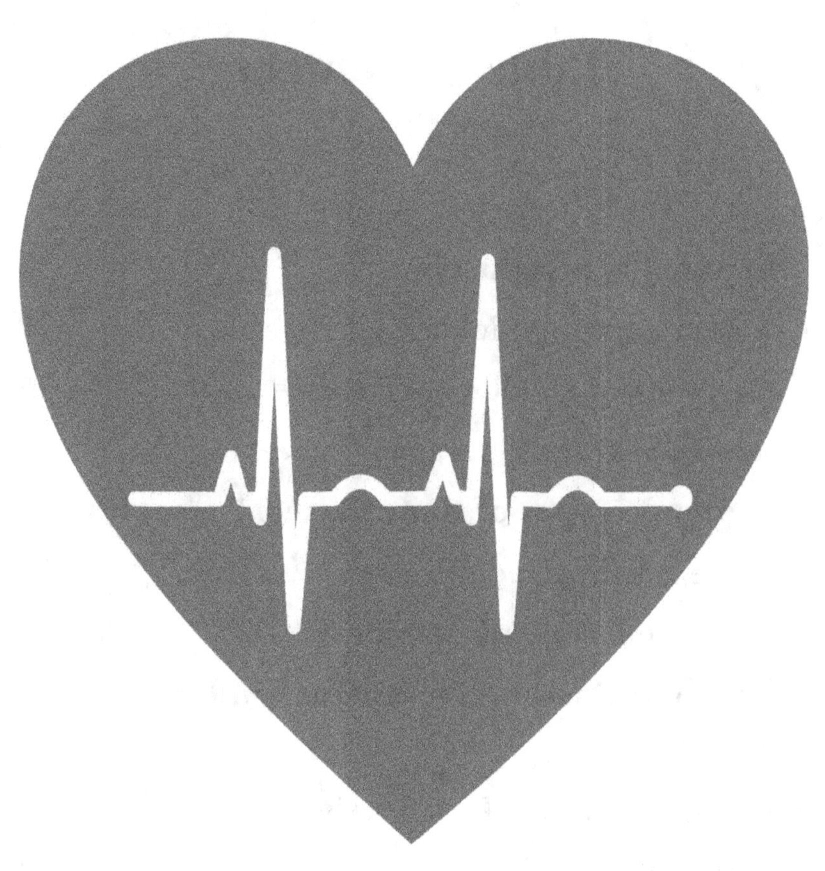

Chapter 1 : Introduction

Sickle cell disease stands as a testament to the resilience of the human spirit in the face of a relentless genetic disorder. For decades, individuals and families grappling with this condition have navigated a path laden with pain, complications, and uncertainty. However, in recent years, a beacon of hope has emerged on the horizon of medical science – gene-based therapy.

This book embarks on a journey through the intricate landscapes of sickle cell disease, exploring the revolutionary prospects offered by gene-based therapies. It endeavors to unravel the complexities of this hereditary ailment, delving into the foundations of genetic science and the transformative potential of emerging treatment modalities.

Understanding Sickle Cell Disease

At its core, sickle cell disease is a genetic condition characterized by the abnormal structure of hemoglobin, the protein responsible for carrying oxygen in red blood cells. This anomaly causes red blood cells to adopt a sickle-like shape, leading to blockages in blood vessels, chronic pain, and organ damage. Understanding the genetic underpinnings of this disease forms the cornerstone of our quest for effective treatments.

The Need for Advanced Treatments

Despite advancements in conventional therapies to manage symptoms, the need for a definitive cure remains paramount. Patients and their families endure the burden of recurrent hospitalizations, pain crises, and limitations on daily life. It is within this context of unmet medical needs that gene-based therapies emerge as a beacon of hope, offering the promise of not just managing but eradicating this chronic condition at its genetic root.

Exploring Gene-Based Therapy

This book traverses the landscape of gene-based therapies, ranging from the fundamental principles of gene editing techniques to the innovative approaches in gene therapy and stem cell transplantation. Through meticulous examination and explanation, it aims to demystify these advanced treatments, presenting the current landscape of research, trials, and breakthroughs in the field.

Charting a Path Forward

As we delve deeper into the realms of gene-based therapy for sickle cell disease, ethical considerations, accessibility, and the broader societal impact of these treatments come into focus. Discussions on the ethical implications of gene editing, equitable access to these groundbreaking therapies, and their potential societal implications are crucial in charting an inclusive and sustainable path forward.

A Call to Action

This book serves as a rallying cry for researchers, healthcare professionals, policymakers, and society at large to unite in the pursuit of a cure for sickle cell disease. It is a testament to our collective determination to alleviate the suffering of millions affected by this condition and to embrace the transformative power of science and compassion.

As we turn the pages of this exploration into gene-based therapy for sickle cell disease, let us embark together on a journey of discovery, hope, and progress toward a future where the burdens of this genetic ailment are but a distant memory.

Understanding Sickle Cell Disease

Sickle cell disease is an inherited genetic disorder caused by a mutation in the hemoglobin gene responsible for producing hemoglobin, the protein in red blood cells that carries oxygen throughout the body. This mutation leads to the production of abnormal hemoglobin known as hemoglobin S (HbS). Inheriting two copies of the mutated gene (one from each parent) results in sickle cell disease. Individuals with one copy of the mutated gene (sickle cell trait) may have some symptoms but generally lead a normal life.

Physiological Changes:
Hemoglobin S causes red blood cells to change shape from their normal round shape to a sickle or crescent shape when oxygen levels are low or under stress. These sickle-shaped cells are less flexible and can stick together, leading to blockages in small blood vessels. This blockage reduces blood flow, causing tissue damage and depriving organs of oxygen, leading to pain, organ damage, and a range of complications.

Clinical Manifestations

Sickle cell disease manifests differently in individuals. Common symptoms include:

Pain Crises: Severe and sudden episodes of pain due to blocked blood flow.

Anemia: The destruction of red blood cells leads to a shortage, causing fatigue and weakness.

Increased Susceptibility to Infections: SCD weakens the immune system, making individuals more susceptible to infections.

Organ Damage: Reduced blood flow can damage various organs, leading to complications like strokes, kidney damage, lung complications, and more.

Delayed Growth: Sickle cell disease can affect children's growth and development.

Complications:

The disease can result in a range of complications, including acute chest syndrome (a life-threatening lung condition), stroke, priapism (painful erection in males), gallstones, and leg ulcers. It can also increase the risk of other health problems, impacting overall quality of life.

Psychosocial Impact:

Beyond the physical aspects, sickle cell disease can impact mental health and social well-being. The unpredictability of pain crises, frequent hospital visits, and limitations in daily activities can lead to stress, anxiety, depression, and difficulties in social interactions, affecting the individual and their family's quality of life.

The Need for Advanced Treatments

The need for advanced treatments in sickle cell disease stems from several critical factors:

Lack of Definitive Cure: Present treatments predominantly focus on symptom management and complications rather than providing a cure for sickle cell disease. Patients endure recurrent pain crises, anemia, and the risk of severe complications without a therapy that addresses the root genetic cause of the condition.

Impact on Quality of Life: Sickle cell disease significantly affects the quality of life of individuals. Chronic pain, frequent hospitalizations, decreased mobility, and limitations in daily activities result in emotional distress and diminished social interactions, impacting both patients and their families.

Healthcare Burden: The disease exerts a substantial economic burden on healthcare systems and families. The costs associated with frequent hospital visits, medication, and interventions for managing complications are high, contributing to healthcare inequalities and financial strain.

Limited Treatment Efficacy: Current treatments like hydroxyurea and blood transfusions have varying degrees of effectiveness and may not be universally accessible or suitable for all patients. There's a need for more efficient and broadly applicable therapies to improve outcomes for all individuals living with sickle cell disease.

Risk of Life-Threatening Complications: Sickle cell disease predisposes individuals to life-threatening complications such as strokes, acute chest syndrome, and infections. Despite medical advancements, these complications remain significant sources of morbidity and mortality in affected individuals.

Pursuit of a Cure: The ultimate goal is to find a cure that can fundamentally alter the disease's course. Advanced treatments, especially gene-based therapies like gene editing and gene therapy, hold promise in addressing the genetic mutation responsible for the production of abnormal hemoglobin, potentially offering a cure or significantly reducing disease severity.

Ethical and Social Considerations: The emergence of gene-based therapies brings ethical considerations regarding accessibility, affordability, and the long-term consequences of genetic interventions. Balancing ethical principles with the imperative to provide equitable access to innovative treatments is a crucial consideration.

In essence, the need for advanced treatments in sickle cell disease arises due to the limitations of current therapies, the immense impact on individuals' lives and healthcare systems, the quest for a definitive cure, and the potential of innovative treatments, particularly gene-based therapies, to revolutionize the management of this inherited genetic disorder. These advanced treatments offer hope for a future where the burden of sickle cell disease can be substantially alleviated or eradicated.

Chapter 2:   Foundations of Gene-Based Therapy

Foundations of Gene-Based Therapy

Gene-based therapy represents a paradigm shift in medical science, leveraging advancements in genetics, molecular biology, and biotechnology to address genetic disorders at their core. In the context of sickle cell disease, understanding the foundations of gene-based therapy is crucial in exploring potential transformative treatments.

Genetics of Sickle Cell Disease

Sickle cell disease results from a specific genetic mutation in the hemoglobin gene, leading to the production of abnormal hemoglobin S (HbS). This genetic alteration causes red blood cells to assume a sickle shape under certain conditions, triggering complications associated with the disease. The foundational understanding of this genetic mutation forms the basis for targeted interventions aimed at correcting or mitigating its effects.

Basics of Gene Therapy

Gene therapy involves the delivery of genetic material into a patient's cells to correct or replace faulty genes. It encompasses various approaches, including gene addition, gene editing, and gene silencing. In the context of sickle cell disease, gene therapy aims to address the underlying genetic defect responsible for the production of abnormal hemoglobin, ultimately restoring the normal function of red blood cells.

Gene Editing Techniques

Technological advancements, particularly CRISPR-Cas9 and other gene editing tools, have revolutionized the field of gene therapy. These techniques enable precise modifications to the DNA sequence, offering the potential to correct the specific mutation causing sickle cell disease. CRISPR-based approaches have shown promise in preclinical studies and early-stage clinical trials for editing the genetic defects associated with the condition.

Stem Cell Transplantation

Stem cell transplantation, particularly hematopoietic stem cell transplantation (HSCT), offers an alternative therapeutic approach. It involves replacing the patient's bone marrow, which produces blood cells, with healthy stem cells from a compatible donor. HSCT has been used as a curative option for some individuals with sickle cell disease, but challenges such as finding suitable donors and the risk of complications limit its widespread applicability.

Understanding these foundational aspects of gene-based therapy lays the groundwork for exploring innovative treatment strategies for sickle cell disease. By targeting the genetic root cause of the condition, these approaches hold the potential to offer curative or significantly disease-modifying interventions that could transform the lives of individuals affected by this inherited blood disorder.

Genetics of Sickle Cell Disease

Sickle cell disease (SCD) is a genetic disorder caused by a specific mutation in the gene that provides instructions for making hemoglobin, the protein in red blood cells responsible for carrying oxygen throughout the body.

Genetic Mutation:

The mutation responsible for sickle cell disease occurs in the HBB gene, which encodes the beta-globin subunit of hemoglobin. In individuals with SCD, a single nucleotide change in the HBB gene results in the substitution of a single amino acid in the beta-globin chain. This change leads to the production of abnormal hemoglobin known as hemoglobin S (HbS).

Hemoglobin S (HbS):

Hemoglobin S differs from normal hemoglobin (hemoglobin A) primarily in its ability to polymerize or stick together when oxygen levels are low. Under conditions of reduced oxygen, HbS molecules can form long, rigid chains within red blood cells, causing the cells to become rigid and assume a characteristic sickle or crescent shape. This change in shape makes the red blood cells less flexible and more prone to getting trapped in small blood vessels, leading to blockages that impair blood flow.

Effects of Abnormal Hemoglobin:

The altered shape of red blood cells due to HbS leads to a range of complications. These include:

Vaso-Occlusive Crises: Sudden and severe episodes of pain occur when sickled red blood cells block blood flow, depriving tissues of oxygen.

Anemia: The lifespan of sickled red blood cells is shorter than that of normal red blood cells, leading to anemia (a reduced number of red blood cells), causing fatigue and weakness.

Organ Damage: Blocked blood flow can damage organs, leading to chronic organ dysfunction or failure.

Increased Susceptibility to Infections: SCD can weaken the immune system, making individuals more prone to infections.

Inheritance Pattern:

Sickle cell disease is inherited in an autosomal recessive pattern. This means that a person must inherit two copies of the mutated HBB gene (one from each parent) to have the disease. If a person inherits one normal copy of the gene and one mutated copy, they will have sickle cell trait, which generally does not cause symptoms but can be passed on to offspring.

Understanding the specific genetic mutation and its effects on hemoglobin production is fundamental in developing targeted therapies aimed at correcting or mitigating the impact of this genetic defect in sickle cell disease.

Basics of Gene Therapy

Gene therapy represents a groundbreaking approach in medicine that involves introducing genetic material into a patient's cells to correct or modify defective genes responsible for diseases. In the context of sickle cell disease (SCD), gene therapy aims to address the underlying genetic mutation that leads to the production of abnormal hemoglobin.

Key Components and Approaches of Gene Therapy:
Gene Addition: In gene addition therapy, functional copies of the defective gene are introduced into the cells to supplement or replace the faulty gene. This can be achieved by delivering the correct gene using viral vectors or non-viral methods into the patient's cells, enabling the production of normal hemoglobin.

Gene Editing: Gene editing technologies like CRISPR-Cas9 allow precise modifications to the DNA sequence. In SCD, gene editing aims to directly correct the specific mutation in the HBB gene responsible for producing abnormal hemoglobin S. By targeting and editing the faulty sequence, the goal is to restore the normal function of hemoglobin, leading to the production of healthy red blood cells.

Gene Silencing: Another approach involves silencing or reducing the expression of the mutated gene responsible for sickle cell disease. This can be accomplished using techniques such as RNA interference (RNAi) or antisense oligonucleotides (ASOs), which target and block the expression of the defective gene, thereby reducing the production of abnormal hemoglobin.

Delivery Systems:

Delivery of therapeutic genetic material into the target cells is a crucial aspect of gene therapy. Various delivery systems are utilized, including:

Viral Vectors: Viruses modified to carry the correct genetic material are used to deliver genes into the patient's cells.

Commonly used viral vectors include adeno-associated viruses (AAVs) and lentiviruses.

Non-viral Vectors: Non-viral methods involve the use of liposomes, nanoparticles, or other non-viral carriers to transport genetic material into cells. These approaches are often less immunogenic but may have lower efficiency compared to viral vectors.

Challenges and Considerations:

Safety: Ensuring the safety of gene therapy interventions is paramount. Concerns include potential off-target effects, immune responses to the therapy, and the possibility of unintended genetic changes.

Efficacy: Achieving sufficient and long-lasting correction of the genetic defect remains a challenge in gene therapy for SCD.

Ethical and Regulatory Considerations: Gene therapy involves manipulation of genetic material, raising ethical concerns regarding the implications of altering human genes and the need for stringent regulatory oversight.

Advancements in gene therapy hold promise for providing potentially curative or disease-modifying treatments for sickle cell disease by targeting the underlying genetic cause. Ongoing research and clinical trials aim to address challenges and further optimize these approaches for safe and effective therapeutic interventions.

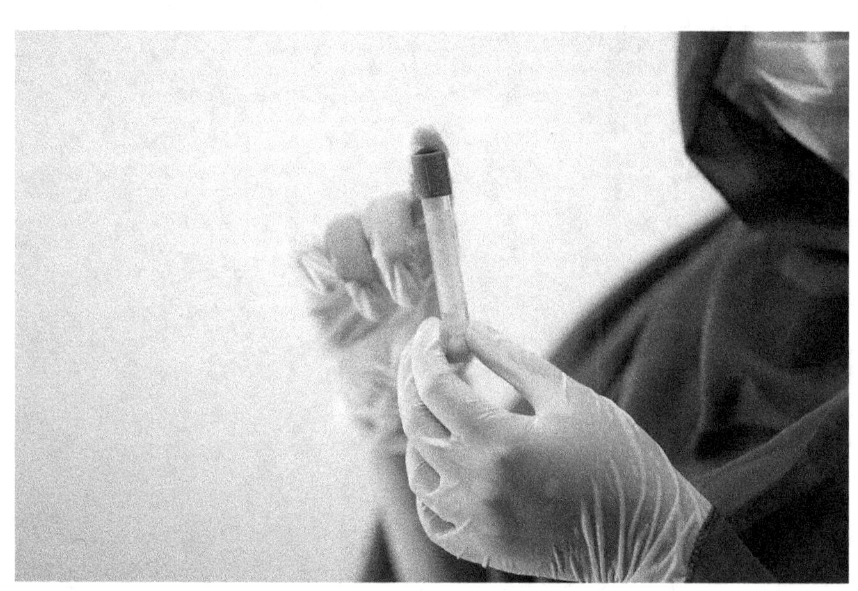

Chapter 3: Types of Gene-Based Therapies

Gene-based therapies encompass various approaches aimed at treating diseases by targeting the underlying genetic abnormalities. In the context of sickle cell disease (SCD), several types of gene-based therapies show promise:

1.   Gene Addition Therapy:

Approach: Introduces functional copies of the correct gene into the patient's cells to compensate for the defective gene responsible for SCD.

Method: Using viral vectors or non-viral methods, the correct gene is delivered into the cells to enable the production of normal hemoglobin, addressing the genetic deficiency causing SCD.

2.   Gene Editing:

Approach: Precisely modifies the DNA sequence to correct the specific mutation in the HBB gene, responsible for producing abnormal hemoglobin S.

Technologies: CRISPR-Cas9 and other gene editing tools target and edit the faulty sequence, aiming to restore the normal function of hemoglobin and the production of healthy red blood cells.

3. Gene Silencing:

Approach: Reduces or silences the expression of the mutated gene responsible for sickle cell disease.

Methods: Utilizes RNA interference (RNAi) or antisense oligonucleotides (ASOs) to target and block the expression of the defective gene, thereby reducing the production of abnormal hemoglobin.

4. Stem Cell Transplantation:

Approach: Replaces the patient's diseased bone marrow with healthy stem cells carrying the correct genetic information.

Method: Hematopoietic stem cell transplantation (HSCT) involves infusing healthy stem cells from a compatible donor into the patient, allowing the production of normal red blood cells.

5. Ex Vivo Gene Therapy:

Approach: Involves modifying the patient's own stem cells outside the body (ex vivo) to correct the genetic defect before reinfusing these modified cells back into the patient.

Procedure: Stem cells are extracted from the patient, genetically modified in a controlled laboratory setting to correct the mutation, and then reintroduced into the patient's body.

Each of these gene-based therapy approaches aims to address the root genetic cause of sickle cell disease by either correcting the defective gene, supplementing it with healthy genes, or reducing the expression of the mutated gene. These innovative strategies hold promise for potentially providing curative or significantly disease-altering treatments for individuals affected by SCD. Ongoing research and clinical trials continue to explore and refine these approaches for safe and effective therapeutic interventions.

Gene Editing Techniques

Gene editing techniques revolutionize the field of genetic therapy by allowing precise modifications to the DNA sequence, thereby correcting specific mutations associated with genetic disorders like sickle cell disease (SCD). Here are some prominent gene editing techniques:

1.   CRISPR-Cas9:

Principle: CRISPR-Cas9 (Clustered Regularly Interspaced Short Palindromic Repeats) is a versatile and widely used gene editing tool derived from the bacterial immune system.

Function: CRISPR-Cas9 functions like molecular scissors, guided by a specifically designed RNA sequence to target a specific location in the DNA. Cas9 enzyme then cleaves the DNA at the targeted site.

Editing Process: After DNA cleavage, the cell's natural repair machinery can introduce changes by either inserting, deleting, or replacing DNA sequences, allowing for precise genetic modifications.

2.   TALENs (Transcription Activator-Like Effector Nucleases):

Design: TALENs are artificial enzymes designed to bind and cut specific DNA sequences.

Mechanism: They are constructed by fusing a DNA-cleaving domain to customizable proteins that bind to specific DNA sequences, allowing for precise DNA cleavage at the targeted site.

3.   ZFNs (Zinc Finger Nucleases):

Structure: ZFNs are engineered proteins comprising a zinc finger DNA-binding domain linked to a DNA-cleaving domain.

Function: The zinc finger domain recognizes and binds to a specific DNA sequence, enabling the attached DNA-cleaving domain to make a precise cut at the targeted site.

4.   Prime Editing:

Novel Technique: Prime editing is a recent advancement in gene editing that combines a modified Cas9 protein with an engineered reverse transcriptase enzyme.

Editing Precision: It allows for precise alterations in the DNA without requiring double-strand breaks, offering increased accuracy in genetic modifications.

5.   Base Editing:

Approach: Base editing is a technique that directly converts one DNA base pair to another without causing double-strand breaks.

Precision: By using engineered fusion proteins, such as CRISPR-Cas9 coupled with a deaminase enzyme, base editing can induce single-letter changes (C to T or A to G) at specific locations in the genome.

Gene editing techniques, particularly CRISPR-Cas9, have garnered significant attention due to their precision, efficiency, and potential for correcting genetic mutations underlying diseases like sickle cell anemia. These tools offer immense promise for developing targeted and potentially curative treatments for genetic disorders by directly addressing the genetic defects at the molecular level. Ongoing research continues to refine these techniques, making them safer and more effective for clinical applications.

Gene Therapy Approaches

Gene therapy encompasses various approaches aimed at treating diseases by manipulating genes or genetic material. In the context of sickle cell disease (SCD), several gene therapy approaches are being explored:

1. Gene Addition Therapy:

Approach: Introduces functional copies of the correct gene into the patient's cells to compensate for the defective gene responsible for SCD.

Delivery Method: Viral vectors, such as adeno-associated viruses (AAVs) or lentiviruses, are commonly used to deliver the correct gene into bone marrow cells or stem cells. These modified cells can then produce normal hemoglobin.

2. Gene Editing:

Approach: Precisely modifies the DNA sequence to correct the specific mutation in the HBB gene, responsible for producing abnormal hemoglobin S.

Technologies: CRISPR-Cas9 and other gene editing tools aim to edit the faulty sequence in hematopoietic stem cells or bone marrow cells, restoring the normal function of hemoglobin and red blood cells.

3. Gene Silencing:

Approach: Reduces or silences the expression of the mutated gene responsible for sickle cell disease.

Methods: Utilizes RNA interference (RNAi) or antisense oligonucleotides (ASOs) to target and block the expression of the defective gene, thereby reducing the production of abnormal hemoglobin.

4. Ex Vivo Gene Therapy:

Approach: Involves modifying the patient's own stem cells outside the body (ex vivo) to correct the genetic defect before reinfusing these modified cells back into the patient.

Procedure: Stem cells are extracted from the patient, genetically modified in a controlled laboratory setting to correct the mutation, and then reintroduced into the patient's body.

5.   In Vivo Gene Therapy:

Approach: Administers therapeutic genes directly into the patient's body.

Delivery Methods: Utilizes viral vectors or non-viral methods to deliver genes to specific tissues or organs affected by sickle cell disease, aiming to correct the genetic defect within the body.

6.   Stem Cell Transplantation with Gene Modification:

Approach: Combines traditional stem cell transplantation with gene modification techniques to replace the patient's bone marrow with genetically modified stem cells.

Procedure: Healthy donor stem cells undergo gene editing before transplantation into the patient, aiming to provide a continuous supply of healthy red blood cells.

Each gene therapy approach offers unique strategies to address the genetic basis of sickle cell disease. These innovative approaches hold promise for potentially providing curative or significantly disease-altering treatments by directly targeting the underlying genetic defects associated with SCD. Ongoing research and clinical trials continue to explore and refine these approaches for safe and effective therapeutic interventions.

Stem Cell Transplantation

Stem cell transplantation, particularly hematopoietic stem cell transplantation (HSCT), is a treatment approach that involves replacing a patient's diseased or malfunctioning bone marrow with healthy stem cells from a compatible donor. In the context of sickle cell disease (SCD), stem cell transplantation aims to provide a source of healthy blood cells that can produce normal hemoglobin, thereby alleviating the symptoms and complications associated with the disease.

Key Elements of Stem Cell Transplantation for SCD:
Hematopoietic Stem Cells (HSCs): These are the precursor cells capable of developing into various types of blood cells, including red blood cells, white blood cells, and platelets. They reside in the bone marrow and are responsible for the continuous production of blood cells throughout life.

Donor Selection: Finding a suitable donor is critical for a successful transplant. Ideally, the donor's tissue type (HLA typing) closely matches that of the recipient to minimize the risk of graft rejection or graft-versus-host disease (GVHD).

Preparation (Conditioning Regimen): Before the transplant, the patient typically undergoes a conditioning regimen involving chemotherapy or radiation therapy. This process aims to suppress the patient's immune system and create space in the bone marrow for the transplanted stem cells.

Transplantation: Healthy stem cells obtained from the donor (usually from bone marrow, peripheral blood, or umbilical cord blood) are infused into the patient's bloodstream through a vein. The transplanted stem cells travel to the bone marrow and gradually begin producing healthy blood cells.

Potential Outcomes and Considerations:

Engraftment: The transplanted stem cells establish themselves in the recipient's bone marrow and start producing healthy blood cells. This process is known as engraftment and can take several weeks to months.

Graft-Versus-Host Disease (GVHD): In some cases, the donor's immune cells may recognize the recipient's body as foreign and attack its tissues. This complication, known as GVHD, can cause various symptoms and requires treatment.

Immune System Recovery: After the transplant, the patient's immune system gradually recovers, and there is a risk of infections until the immune system is fully functional.

Stem cell transplantation, while potentially curative, has limitations, including finding a suitable donor match, risks associated with the procedure (such as GVHD and infections), and the need for extensive pre-transplant preparations. Advances in gene editing and stem cell technologies aim to improve the outcomes and accessibility of stem cell transplantation for sickle cell disease, offering hope for a cure or significant disease improvement in affected individuals.

Chaoter 4: Current Treatments and Limitations

Casgevy

For individuals with sickle cell disease who have repeated vaso-occlusive crises and are 12 years of age or older, the cell-based gene therapy casgevy is licenced. The first treatment using CRISPR/Cas9, a kind of genome editing technology, to receive FDA approval is called Casgevy.

Hematopoietic (blood) stem cells from patients are altered by CRISPR/Cas9 genome editing.

Targeted DNA snipping with CRISPR/Cas9 allows precise editing (removal, insertion, or replacement) of the targeted DNA. After being reintroduced into the patient, the altered blood stem cells engraft—that is, grow within the bone marrow—and boost the synthesis of foetal haemoglobin (HbF), a kind of haemoglobin that helps carry oxygen. Elevated HbF levels stop red blood cells from sickling in sickle cell disease patients.

Information Backing Casgevy

In an ongoing single-arm, multicenter trial, adult and adolescent SCD patients' safety and efficacy were assessed with Casgevy. Prior to screening, at least two severe VOCs as defined by the procedure had been reported by the patients in the two years before. Throughout the 24-month follow-up period, the main effectiveness outcome was the absence of severe VOC episodes for at least 12 months in a row. Casgevy was administered to treat 44 individuals in total. 29 (93.5%) of the 31 patients who had enough follow-up time to be evaluated had this result. No patient had graft failure or rejection; all treated patients underwent effective engraftment.

Low platelet and white blood cell counts, mouth sores, nausea, musculoskeletal discomfort, abdominal pain, vomiting, febrile neutropenia (fever with low white blood cell count), headache, and itching were the most frequent adverse effects.

Lyfgenia

A cell-based gene treatment is called Lyfgenia. Patients 12 years of age and older with sickle cell disease and a history of vaso-occlusive episodes can receive Lyfgenia treatment. Lyfgenia uses a lentiviral vector (gene delivery vehicle) for genetic alteration. The patient's blood stem cells are genetically altered to create HbAT87Q, a haemoglobin derived via gene therapy that works similarly to haemoglobin A, the typical adult haemoglobin produced in people without sickle cell disease, in the case of Lyfgenia. The likelihood of sickling and obstructing blood flow is reduced in red blood cells carrying HbAT87Q. The patient receives these altered stem cells after that.

In hematopoietic stem cell transplantation, both products are created from the patient's transformed blood stem cells, which are administered as a single-use, one-dose infusion. Before beginning treatment, the patient's own stem cells are extracted. Next, the patient has to have high-dose chemotherapy, or myeloablative conditioning, which eliminates bone marrow cells in order to replace them with the altered cells found in Casgevy and Lyfgenia. A long-term research will be conducted to assess the safety and efficacy of Lyfgenia and Casgevy in patients who received them.

Information for Lyfgenia

Based on data analysis from a single-arm, 24-month multicenter research involving individuals with sickle cell disease and a history of VOEs between the ages of 12- and 50, Lyfgenia's safety and efficacy have been determined. The full resolution of VOEs (VOE-CR) between 6 and 18 months following Lyfgenia infusion was used to measure the effectiveness. During this time, 28 (88%) out of 32 patients obtained VOE-CR.

The most frequent side effects, which were consistent with chemotherapy and underlying disease, were febrile neutropenia (fever and low white blood cell count), low levels of platelets, white blood cells, and red blood cells, and stomatitis (mouth sores of the lips, mouth, and neck).

Hematologic malignancy, or blood cancer, has happened to Lyfgenia-treated patients. On the label of Lyfgenia, there is a black box warning that details this risk. Patients who use this medicine should have ongoing cancer screenings for the rest of their lives.

Applications for Casgevy and Lyfgenia were given the following designations: Orphan Drug, Fast Track, Regenerative Medicine Advanced Therapy, and Priority Review.

The FDA approved Lyfgenia for Bluebird Bio Inc. and Casgevy for Vertex Pharmaceuticals Inc.

Chapter 5: Future Perspectives

The future perspective for a cure for sickle cell disease (SCD) appears promising due to ongoing advancements in various therapeutic approaches, particularly in gene-based therapies. Here are some aspects contributing to the optimistic outlook:

Gene Editing and Gene Therapy Advancements: Techniques like CRISPR-Cas9 and other gene editing tools hold immense potential for precisely targeting and correcting the genetic mutation responsible for SCD. Clinical trials focusing on these innovative approaches have shown promising results in preclinical studies and early-stage human trials.

Advances in Stem Cell Technology: Stem cell transplantation, combined with gene editing or modification techniques, continues to evolve. Researchers are exploring ways to improve the safety, efficacy, and accessibility of stem cell transplantation as a potential curative treatment for SCD.

Ex Vivo Gene Therapy: Modifying a patient's own stem cells outside the body (ex vivo) to correct the genetic defect before reinfusing these modified cells back into the patient holds promise. Continued research aims to refine this approach to ensure the sustained production of healthy red blood cells.

Clinical Trials and Therapeutic Innovation: Ongoing clinical trials focusing on gene-based therapies, including gene editing, gene addition, and gene silencing techniques, are progressing. These trials aim to assess the safety, efficacy, and long-term outcomes of these advanced therapies in treating SCD.

Collaborative Research Efforts: Collaboration between researchers, clinicians, biotech companies, and pharmaceutical firms plays a crucial role in accelerating therapeutic development. International collaboration and increased funding for SCD research further facilitate the exploration of potential cures and improved treatments.

Precision Medicine Approaches: Advances in understanding the individual variability in SCD, including its diverse clinical manifestations, genetic modifiers, and response to treatments, pave the way for personalized therapeutic approaches tailored to each patient's specific needs.

While the journey toward a definitive cure for sickle cell disease continues, the landscape of SCD treatment is witnessing rapid advancements, offering hope for a future where individuals affected by this genetic disorder may have access to curative therapies. However, challenges such as ensuring safety, scalability, accessibility, and ethical considerations remain critical factors in the development and implementation of these potential cures. Ongoing research and clinical trials are key in realizing the vision of a cure and significantly improving the lives of those affected by SCD.

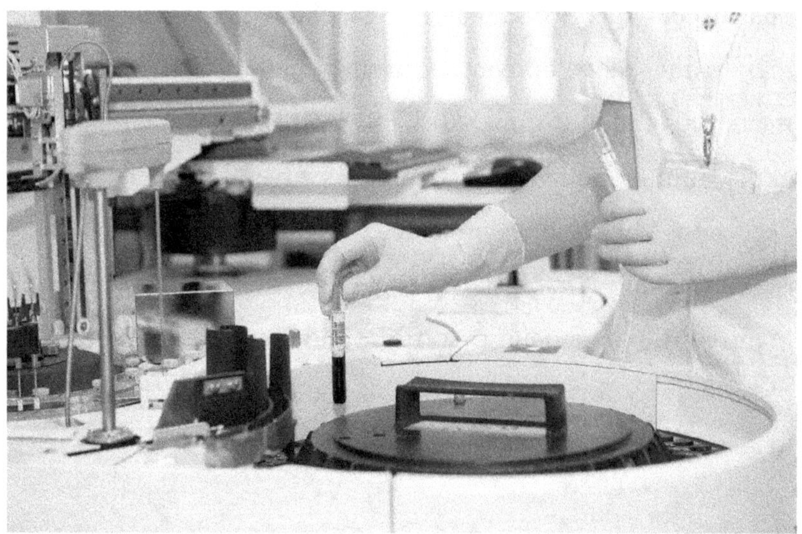

Chapter 6: Conclusion

In conclusion, the pursuit of a definitive cure for sickle cell disease (SCD) stands at an encouraging juncture, thanks to remarkable advancements in gene-based therapies, particularly gene editing, gene addition, and gene silencing techniques. These innovative approaches hold promise in directly targeting the genetic root cause of SCD, offering potential curative or disease-modifying treatments. Ongoing research, clinical trials, and collaborative efforts among scientists, clinicians, and pharmaceutical entities underscore a collective dedication to advancing therapeutic options for SCD.

The evolution of precision medicine, personalized treatments, and refinements in stem cell technologies also contribute to the optimistic outlook for improved interventions tailored to individual patient needs. However, while substantial progress has been made, challenges persist, including ensuring the safety, efficacy, scalability, and equitable accessibility of these emerging therapies.

The future perspective for a cure or transformative treatments for SCD remains bright, driven by relentless scientific exploration, innovative therapeutic strategies, and a commitment to alleviating the burdens faced by individuals affected by this inherited blood disorder. Continued research endeavors, ethical considerations, and sustained collaborations hold the key to realizing the vision of eradicating SCD and significantly enhancing the lives of millions impacted by this condition worldwide.

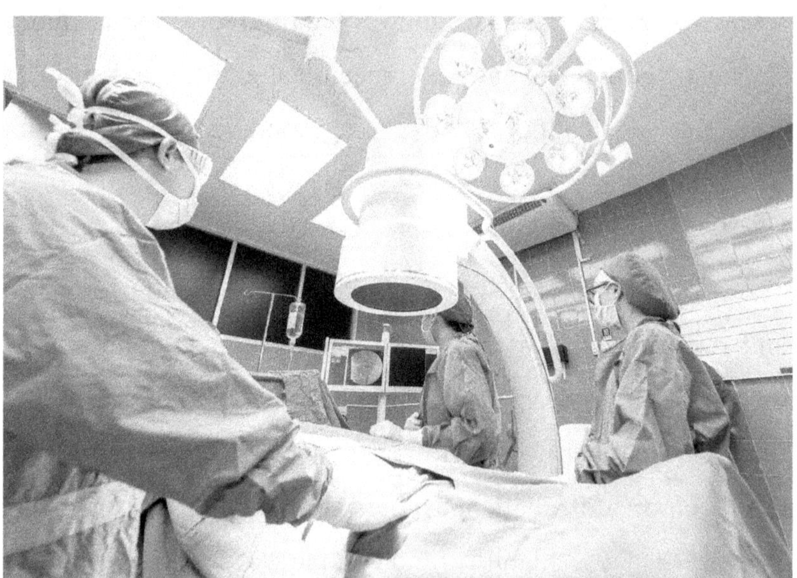